Navigating Perimenopause Challenges

The Complete Guide to Managing Perimenopause

Joy Harry

By reading this document, the reader agrees that under no circumstances is the author responsible for any losses, direct or indirect, that are incurred as a result of the use of the information contained within this document, including, but not limited to, errors, omissions, or inaccuracies.

Table of Contents

Table of Contents

Acknowledgments

Introduction

Chapter 1: Physical Challenges

Hormonal Fluctuations and Their Effects

Irregular Menstrual Cycles

Increased Menstrual Cramping and Heavy Bleeding

Hot Flashes and Night Sweats

Sleep Disturbances

Insomnia During Perimenopause

Fatigue During Perimenopause

Impact of Sleep Deprivation on Daily Life

Changes in Mood and Libido

Anxiety, Depression, and Mood Swings

Estrogen and Its Role in Mood Regulation

Progesterone and Its Calming Effect

Decreased Sexual Desire and Painful Intercourse

Biological Factors

Psychological Factors

Social Factors

Chapter 2: Emotional Challenges

Coping with Uncertainty and Loss of Control

Dealing With Unpredictable Symptoms

Grieving the Loss of Reproductive Ability

Emotional Impact

Biological and Social Factors

Personal Narratives and Identity

Impact on Mental Health

Biological Factors

Psychological Stress

Increased Vulnerability

Symptoms and Diagnosis

Impact on Daily Life

Feeling Overwhelmed and Unable to Cope

Importance of Emotional Support

Emotional Stability and Mental Health

Strengthening Relationships

Validation and Normalization of Experiences

Encouragement and Motivation

Access to Resources and Information

Chapter 3: Social Challenges

Interpersonal Relationships

Partner Relationships

Social and Workplace Relationships

Family Dynamics

Professional Life

Challenges in the Workplace

    Cognitive and Physical Symptoms

    Workplace Environment

    Discrimination and Bias

    Mental Health Impact

Considering Career Changes or Early Retirement

    Physical and Cognitive Demands

    Emotional and Psychological Impact

    Workplace Environment

    Reevaluating Priorities

    Financial Considerations

Societal Attitudes Towards Aging and Perimenopause

    Ageism and Gender Stereotypes

    Lack of Awareness and Understanding

    Cultural Norms and Expectations

    Media Representation

Internalized Ageism and Shame

    Understanding Internalized Ageism

    What Women See Affects Them

    Shame and Its Impact

Importance of Raising Awareness and Promoting Understanding

    Bridging Knowledge Gaps

    Fostering Empathy and Support

    Improving Healthcare and Workplace Environments

Addressing Societal Attitudes and Stereotypes

Enhancing Research and Policy Development

Chapter 4: Seeking Help and Finding Solutions

Why Should A Woman Seek Help?

Professional Expertise

Emotional and Psychological Benefits

Improved Quality of Life

Prevention of Complications

Empowerment and Self-Efficacy

Importance of Open Communication with Healthcare Providers

Ensuring Accurate Diagnosis

Tailoring Treatment Plans

Addressing Concerns and Preferences

Managing Expectations and Education

Building a Supportive Relationship

Monitoring and Adjusting Treatment

Navigating Complex Health Issues

Hormone Replacement Therapy and Other Medical Options

Hormone Replacement Therapy (HRT)

Types of HRT

Risks and Considerations

Non-Hormonal Medical Options

Alternative Therapies

Monitoring and Adjusting Treatment

Lifestyle Modifications

    Diet and Nutrition

    Exercise and Physical Activity

    Sleep and Rest

    Identify and Avoid Triggers

    Stress Management Techniques

        Mindfulness and Meditation

        Deep Breathing Exercises

        Progressive Muscle Relaxation

        Time Management and Organization

        Creative Outlets

  Support Groups and Therapy

    Benefits of Support Groups

    Types of Therapy

Conclusion

Glossary

References

Acknowledgments

To every woman who may have suffered from perimenopause, and to every woman who may have trouble in the future, know that there is help. I don't want you to feel as though you are alone on this journey. You are not alone; you have not gone unnoticed! I hope that every woman who reads this will find comfort in knowing they are not crazy, and life will get better. Thank you to everyone who has been an inspiration and supported me along the journey through the last three years!

Introduction

Did you know that according to research, almost 6,000 women in the United States reach perimenopause every day, translating to more than two million women annually? (Shiramizu, 2024). Perimenopause is an important and universal experience that impacts millions of women worldwide.

Perimenopause, also referred to as menopausal transition, is a natural transition period that usually occurs in a woman's life during their 40s, but sometimes can begin as early as the mid-30s or as late as the early 50s (WebMD Editorial Contributors, 2023). This transitional phase marks a slow decline in ovarian function that further leads up to menopause. This decline is quite erratic, leading to irregular and varying menstrual cycles and symptoms commonly linked with perimenopause. During perimenopause, hormonal fluctuations—especially the levels of progesterone and estrogen—cause a range of symptoms that can last from many months to many years (usually between four to ten years). It ends one year after the last menstrual period, which foreshadows the official onset of menopause.

The time of perimenopause not only precedes menopause, but a large portion of the female population experiences challenges with this change or its symptoms at some point in their lives. This can vary greatly based on factors like lifestyle, genetics, and overall well-being. For example, women who have undergone some medical treatments, such as chemotherapy, or who smoke regularly, can experience an earlier onset of perimenopause.

Understanding the challenges of perimenopause is vital for a number of reasons. Welcome to *Navigating Perimenopause Challenges*, where we will not only learn about the challenges but also strategies to deal with this transition.

But first, let us understand the difference between perimenopause and premenopause. Although they may sound the same, they are quite different. Generally, premenopause refers to the whole period of a woman's reproductive life before the beginning of perimenopause. However, it is occasionally used to define the phase just before perimenopause starts. Perimenopause, on the other hand, is when a woman transitions into menopause.

When you know about something, it significantly reduces your anxiety associated with the unknown. Likewise, understanding the challenges of perimenopause helps in normalizing the experience and minimizing the stigma that typically surrounds discussions of perimenopause as well as aging. There are many women who feel embarrassed or isolated by their symptoms during this phase, but awareness can facilitate a supportive environment where they feel heard, validated, and understood. This supportive environment becomes a platform where you can share your experiences and seek professional help.

Know that perimenopause offers a unique set of emotional, physical, and social challenges that can impact your quality of life. Identifying the emotional, physical, and social effects of perimenopause allows you to seek appropriate medical advice and treatments. We will also talk about these challenges in detail in the upcoming chapters. Here we will have a glimpse of these challenges:

- **Hot flashes and night sweats:** One of the most common symptoms is hot flashes. Experiencing sudden feelings of extreme heat can cause you discomfort and sweating. Night sweats, the nighttime version of hot flashes, can disrupt sleep and contribute to persistent fatigue.

- **Irregular periods:** As hormone levels change, menstrual cycles become very unpredictable. Periods may become lighter or heavier, shorter or longer, and the interval between periods can also change.

- **Sleep disturbances:** Hormonal changes can induce insomnia or frequent waking during the night, leading to daytime irritability and fatigue.

- **Vaginal dryness and sexual discomfort:** Minimized estrogen levels can cause thinning as well as drying of the vaginal tissues, leading to discomfort during intercourse and multiplying the risk of infections.

- **Weight gain and metabolic changes:** Hormonal shifts can impact metabolism, resulting in weight gain, particularly around the abdomen, and enhancing the risk of metabolic syndrome along with cardiovascular diseases.

By acknowledging these issues, your healthcare provider can give you effective management strategies, such as hormone therapy, lifestyle modifications, and alternative treatments.

Perimenopause can also have deep psychological and emotional effects. Hormonal fluctuations can impact your mood and mental health, leading to:

- **Mood swings:** Women can experience rapid mood changes, from anxiety and irritability to depression and sadness.

- **Memory and concentration issues:** Cognitive changes, often known as "brain fog," can affect concentration, memory, and overall mental clarity.

- **Increased stress and anxiety:** The physical symptoms of perimenopause, infused with life stressors, such as family responsibilities and career demands can lead to heightened stress and anxiety levels.

Ultimately, understanding perimenopause helps in promoting overall health and quality of life. The hormonal changes during this time can also enhance the risk of certain health conditions, like cardiovascular disease and osteoporosis (WebMD Editorial Contributors, 2023). It is by being informed about these risks that you can take proactive steps to mitigate them through exercise, diet, and regular medical check-ups.

Throughout a woman's life, she lacks a more inclusive and accepting view of aging, urging them to conceal this phase from society rather than celebrating the wisdom and experience that come with it.

In the upcoming chapters, we will learn about all the challenges that may cause you discomfort and look at the coping strategies so that you may navigate this phase with ease and comfort.

So, get ready to enjoy this period to the fullest!

Chapter 1: Physical Challenges

"I'm not the energetic, outgoing person I used to be. I've lost my fun side. I'm moody, irritable, angry, and sad. And on certain days I have all of those emotions within 10 minutes!" - Daniel Goleman

Perimenopause foreshadows the arrival of a range of physical challenges, including increased menstrual cramping and heavy bleeding, irregular menstrual cycles, hot flashes, and night sweats. Understanding these symptoms and their underlying causes can empower you to seek appropriate treatments and make lifestyle adjustments to manage all these symptoms effectively. In this chapter, we will learn about these physical challenges in detail.

Hormonal Fluctuations and Their Effects

Let's meet Sarah. She is a 45-year-old graphic designer who noticed her once-predictable periods becoming quite irregular. Some months she would skip her period completely, while other months her menstrual cycle would last for merely 21 days rather than her usual 28. This unpredictability took a toll on her mental health and made it tough for her to plan her life around her menstrual cycle which, in turn, affected her social activities and work.

Irregular Menstrual Cycles

During perimenopause, one of the most common changes you will experience is irregular menstrual cycles. This is mainly due to the erratic changes in estrogen and progesterone levels. The ovaries start releasing these hormones inconsistently, which then disrupts the regularity of menstrual cycles (WebMD Editorial Contributors, 2023).

Irregular menstrual cycles during perimenopause can appear in several ways:

- **Skipped periods:** Women can experience skipped periods for one or more months due to diminished ovarian function. This is sometimes one of the first signs of perimenopause.

- **Shorter or longer cycles:** Hormonal imbalances can also cause the menstrual cycle to lengthen or shorten. Rather than a regular 28-day cycle, some women can experience cycles as short as 21 days or as long as 35 days (oligomenorrhea).

- **Changes in flow:** The flow of menstrual blood can also fluctuate. Some women have lighter periods, while others may experience very heavy periods.

Increased Menstrual Cramping and Heavy Bleeding

As hormone levels change, many women endure enhanced menstrual cramping and heavier bleeding during perimenopause (Shiramizu, 2024). These symptoms are the result of an imbalance between two hormones, resulting in the thickening of the uterine lining and more severe uterine contractions.

There are many reasons why menstrual cramping and heavy bleeding (menorrhagia) occur during perimenopause, such as:

1. **Endometrial hyperplasia:** Varying estrogen levels can force the endometrium (the lining of the uterus) to grow thicker than normal which results in heavy menstrual bleeding (Chisholm, 2023).

2. **Uterine fibroids:** These start growths in the uterus, which are very common in women in their 40s and 50s, and can cause both enhanced cramping and heavy bleeding (Chisholm, 2023).

3. **Adenomyosis:** This is the condition where the inner lining of the uterus breaks through the muscle wall of the uterus and causes severe cramping and heavy periods (Chisholm, 2023).

Hot Flashes and Night Sweats

Jane is a 47-year-old financial analyst who experienced frequent hot flashes that left her feeling entirely flushed and sweaty, sometimes many times a day. These episodes were extremely embarrassing during meetings at work. At night, she would frequently wake up drenched in sweat, experiencing sleep disturbances and daytime fatigue.

Hot flashes and night sweats are among the most disruptive and common symptoms of perimenopause. These symptoms arise from your body's response to declining estrogen levels, which influence the hypothalamus- the brain part that is responsible for regulating body temperature (Schulman, 2023).

Hot flashes generally occur as a sudden feeling of heat that spreads through your upper body, sometimes followed by sweating and redness. Night sweats are specifically hot flashes that present when you are sleeping, leading to excessive sweating that can easily soak through bedding and sleepwear.

Several factors can initiate or further exacerbate hot flashes as well as night sweats:

- **Stress:** Emotional stress can activate the hypothalamus to misinterpret body temperature, resulting in hot flashes (WebMD Editorial Contributors, 2023).

- **Diet:** Spicy foods, alcohol, and caffeine can trigger hot flashes in many women.

- **Environmental factors:** Hot weather, heavy bedding, and warm rooms can also lead to the frequency and severity of these symptoms (WebMD Editorial Contributors, 2023).

Sleep Disturbances

Sleep disturbances are a noticeable concern for many women undergoing perimenopause. Hormonal shifts during this transitional phase can easily disrupt normal sleep patterns, contributing to persistent fatigue and insomnia.

Insomnia During Perimenopause

Insomnia is a sleep condition marked by difficulty falling asleep, waking up too early, or difficulty staying asleep. It is a very common issue during perimenopause. The instability in hormone levels, particularly progesterone and estrogen, plays an important role in these sleep disturbances. Estrogen impacts the regulation of neurotransmitters that affect sleep, while progesterone has a soothing effect that aids in sleep initiation (Lee et al., 2019).

But what are neurotransmitters? Neurotransmitters are chemicals that can transmit signals in the brain and play a main role in regulating emotions, mood, and cognitive functions.

Let us meet Lisa, a 46-year-old nurse. She found herself struggling to fall asleep at night. In spite of feeling exhausted and tired, she would lie awake for several hours, unable to silence her thoughts. Her sleep disruptions were further accompanied by night sweats, which led her to wake up uncomfortable and drenched.

Insomnia during perimenopause can be triggered by several factors:

1. **Hormonal fluctuations:** The erratic levels of progesterone and estrogen can easily interfere with your body's natural sleep-wake cycle. Estrogen's role in maintaining sleep quality becomes compromised, leading to unusual awakenings during the night.

2. **Hot flashes:** As discussed earlier, hot flashes and night sweats can cause disruption in sleep. The sudden rush of sweating and heat can make it hard for you to stay asleep or return to sleep after waking up.

3. **Anxiety and stress:** Hormonal changes can multiply anxiety and stress levels, which can lead to difficulty falling asleep and maintaining sleep peacefully throughout the night.

Fatigue During Perimenopause

persistent fatigue is another common issue associated with sleep disturbances during perimenopause. When sleep is regularly interrupted or of poor quality, it results in a cumulative outcome of exhaustion that has the potential to disrupt your daily life. Fatigue during perimenopause is more than feeling tired; it is also about not having clear mental clarity, emotional stability, and compromised physical health.

Impact of Sleep Deprivation on Daily Life

The results of sleep deprivation during perimenopause extend far beyond simply making you tired. persistent sleep disturbances can greatly impact several aspects of day-to-day life, like physical health, emotional well-being, social interactions, and cognitive function.

1. Physical health

Sleep deprivation can have major implications on your physical health. Prolonged lack of sleep has been associated with a range of health issues, such as:

- **Weakened immune system:** Prolonged sleep disturbances can compromise the immune system, making you more susceptible to illnesses and infections (Kong et al., 2023).

- **Increased risk of persistent conditions:** Continuous sleep issues can lead to the development of persistent conditions, such as diabetes, hypertension, and cardiovascular diseases (Kong et al., 2023).

- **Weight gain:** Sleep deprivation can influence hormonal balance linked with appetite and hunger, potentially leading to weight gain and obesity.

Take the example of Ellen, a 50-year-old woman who realized that her sleep disturbances were starting to impact her physical well-being. She found herself catching colds repeatedly and struggled to maintain her blood pressure, which had been well-controlled before. Her fatigue also cultivated an increased craving for sugary snacks. As a result, she gained a lot of weight.

2. Cognitive function

persistent sleep deprivation can impair cognitive functions such as memory, focus, and decision-making skills (Kong et al., 2023). During perimenopause, when cognitive changes may already be taking place, sleep disturbances can aggravate these issues, making daily tasks and responsibilities tougher to deal with.

3. Emotional well-being

Sleep disturbances can also affect your emotional well-being. persistent lack of sleep is paired with mood disorders, such as anxiety and depression, which can be multiplied by the hormonal changes of perimenopause (Kong et al., 2023).

For example, if you are facing increasing mood swings and severe feelings of depression, insomnia can lead to heightened irritability and a decreased ability to cope with everyday stressors. The lack of quality sleep can also give you a sense of frustration and hopelessness.

4. Social and relationship impact

Additionally, sleep deprivation can strain your social relationships and social interactions. The mood swings and irritability resulting from persistent fatigue can give birth to conflicts or arguments with your friends, family members, and colleagues. The decreased energy levels can minimize social engagement along with enjoyment. You may not be inclined toward participating in social activities. Changing moods can also make it easier to misinterpret a conveyed message. Simply put, misunderstanding starts to affect your relationships.

5. Professional impact

Lack of sleep can also affect your career prospects and job performance. Reduced productivity, enhanced absenteeism (you regularly stay away from work without any good reason), and compromised problem-solving abilities can affect your performance.

For example, you may have trouble meeting deadlines and find yourself making errors in your reports. Fatigue and minimized concentration may cause you to fall behind on projects further affecting your professional reputation.

Changes in Mood and Libido

You might not have known until now that mood changes during perimenopause are nothing less than a rollercoaster ride. Sometimes, increased anxiety knocks on your door, other times, you let depression embrace you. Then there are some fleeting moments of joy. Let us understand these mood changes to address the emotional challenges of perimenopause and enhance the overall quality of life.

Anxiety, Depression, and Mood Swings

The psychological symptoms can be as distressing as the physical alterations women experience during perimenopause.

- *Anxiety* is marked by persistent nervousness, fear, or worry that can interfere with your everyday activities or tasks. Research has indicated that women with a history of anxiety or other mental health illnesses are particularly more vulnerable during this time (Alblooshi et al., 2023).

- *Depression* entails prolonged periods of hopelessness, sadness, and a lack of interest in activities that you once enjoyed. The risk of depression can be enhanced two to three times during the perimenopausal phase. Besides this, life stressors common during midlife, such as caring for aging parents or dealing with children leaving home, can compound feelings of depression (Alblooshi et al., 2023).

- *Mood swings* refer to extreme and rapid changes in your emotional state, often without a clear cause.

The hormonal changes during perimenopause are a key driver of these mood changes Hormones that regulate the menstrual cycle also largely affect neurotransmitter activity in the brain, including dopamine and serotonin, which are required for mood regulation.

Estrogen is a key hormone in the female body that influences mood through its impact on neurotransmitters in the brain.

Estrogen and Its Role in Mood Regulation

1. **Serotonin:** Estrogen influences serotonin, a neurotransmitter also known as the "feel-good" chemical. Serotonin levels control appetite, sleep, and mood. Estrogen helps in the regulation of serotonin synthesis and receptor activity, which leads to a balanced mood (Cherry, 2021). When estrogen levels decrease, as they do during perimenopause, serotonin levels also fluctuate, potentially contributing to symptoms of anxiety and depression.

2. **Dopamine:** Estrogen also affects dopamine, another neurotransmitter involved in reward processing and mood regulation. Dopamine leads to feelings of motivation and pleasure (Cherry, 2021). Low estrogen levels can cause disruption in dopamine production, impacting emotional well-being and leading to feeling lack of motivation or sadness.

Progesterone and Its Calming Effect

Progesterone is another main hormone that has a calming effect on the body and brain. It is important for its function in preparing the uterus for pregnancy and regulating the menstrual cycle. This hormone also has a sedative effect, which helps with relaxation and sleep.

1. **Calming effects:** It helps to counterbalance the stimulating effects of estrogen. During perimenopause, as progesterone levels drop, the lack of this calming and soothing effect can worsen feelings of irritability and anxiety (Cherry, 2021). You may find it harder to calm down and may experience heightened emotional volatility and stress.

2. **Sleep and mood:** Progesterone also contributes to sleep quality, which is tied to mood regulation. As progesterone levels decrease, you may experience insomnia, constant fatigue, and exacerbating mood swings and depressive thoughts.

Decreased Sexual Desire and Painful Intercourse

Libido is also known as sex drive or sexual desire. It can be defined as having an interest or inclination to sexual activity. In women, libido is affected by a complex interplay of biological, psychological, and social factors.

Biological Factors

As estrogen and progesterone are the main hormones associated with the menstrual cycle, they also affect sexual desire. Estrogen usually increases libido, while progesterone can have a suppressive effect. Testosterone is present in smaller amounts in females compared to males but it is also vital for maintaining sexual desire. Furthermore, neurotransmitters, such as dopamine and serotonin also influence libido levels. Dopamine stimulates sexual arousal and desire, while serotonin can impede it (Cappelletti & Wallen, 2016). Changes in these hormone levels during different life phases, such as pregnancy, puberty, postpartum, and perimenopause, can greatly increase or decrease libido.

Psychological Factors

Mental health and emotional well-being are essential determinants of female libido. Stress depression, and low self-esteem can lower sexual desire. Contrarily, good self-image positive emotional states, and healthy relationships can increase libido. Psychological factors also entail previous sexual experiences and trauma, which can deeply influence current sexual desire and functioning. Libido can also be influenced by cognitive aspects, such as thoughts, fantasies, and the ability to be present and mindful during sexual activity.

Social Factors

Societal, cultural, and relational aspects also play important roles. Societal attitudes toward cultural norms, sex, and upbringing can shape a woman's libido. For example, in societies where sexuality is taboo or stigmatized, women may experience lower libido. On the other hand, positive and open discussions about sexuality can increase sexual desire. Relationship dynamics, including emotional intimacy, communication, and overall satisfaction, are important too. A good and understanding partner can positively impact libido, while relationship conflicts combined with a lack of emotional connection can decrease sexual desire.

Decreased sexual desire, also referred to as *hypoactive sexual desire disorder* (HSDD), is marked by a lack of interest in sexual activity that results in personal distress. *Dyspareunia* refers to recurrent or persistent genital pain that happens just before, during, or after intercourse.

According to recent studies, more than 50% of women experience decreased sexual desire in this stage (Bostani Khalesi et al., 2020). Similarly, painful intercourse affects about 17-45% of women during perimenopause (Wiginton, 2024).

There are many psychological and physiological factors that contribute to changes in libido and sexual function during perimenopause. Some are:

- **Hormonal changes:** Diminishing levels of estrogen can result in vaginal dryness and thinning of the vaginal walls (vaginal atrophy), which can make intercourse very painful and decrease sexual desire. The reduced production of estrogen and testosterone hormones lowers libido. As a result, you may not show an inclination toward sex. It can strain your relationships and damage your self-esteem.

- **Testosterone:** Although mainly known as a male hormone, testosterone also plays a part in female sexual desire. During perimenopause, levels of testosterone can drop, contributing to a decreased libido.

- **Psychological factors:** Anxiety, stress, and depression can also greatly impact sexual desire as well as enjoyment. Concerns about body image, relationship problems, and overall well-being can lessen sexual interest.

As you have understood the physical challenges, let's move on to the emotional challenges in the next chapter.

Chapter 2: Emotional Challenges

Our feelings are not there to be cast out or conquered. They're there to be engaged and expressed with imagination and intelligence. -T.K. Coleman

Perimenopause can be as emotionally challenging as it is physically. A lot of women undergo a sense of loss of control, grieve the loss of reproductive ability, and feel uncertain most of the time. This chapter is dedicated to learning all about how the emotional world is affected in this important phase of life.

Coping with Uncertainty and Loss of Control

Like many other women, you may experience a sense of constant uncertainty and loss of control over your emotions and body.

One main source of uncertainty during perimenopause is the unpredictability of menstrual cycles. Hormonal fluctuations cause periods to become irregular, which, in turn, can make it hard to predict and manage your menstrual symptoms. This adds to the sense of instability.

Another major factor contributing to feelings of loss of control is multiple physical symptoms resulting from perimenopause. Hot flashes, sleep disturbances, and night sweats impact daily life and take a toll on emotional well-being as well. Emotional changes become prevalent during this phase, therefore, women suffer a sense of uncertainty.

You may experience mood swings, increased irritation, and elevated anxiety. Although these emotional shifts are associated with hormonal changes, they can also be aggravated by the stress of managing all such physical symptoms in this part of life. The unpredictability of these emotional transitions can make it difficult for many women to feel in control of their own mental and emotional state.

Besides the emotional and physical symptoms, perimenopause can bring about changes in sexual function and libido as discussed in the previous chapter. Reduced estrogen levels lead to vaginal dryness and discomfort during intercourse, which can easily affect intimate relationships. The influence on sexual health can be very distressing and give rise to feelings of either frustration or inadequacy, further lowering the sense of control over your own body.

Likewise, perimenopause can affect a woman's confidence and self-image. For example, when you start to observe your physical changes, such as thinning hair, skin changes, and weight gain, they alter your perception regarding your own vitality and attractiveness. This shift in self-image can erode your confidence and further exacerbate the emotional turmoil you are experiencing during this time.

It is also very helpful to consider the social as well as cultural context in which perimenopause occurs. Societal attitudes toward aging and perimenopause can shape how you not only perceive but also cope with this transition. In many cultures, perimenopause is seen positively as a time of enhanced wisdom followed by freedom, while in others, it may be stigmatized and linked with the loss of femininity. These cultural attitudes, as a result, force women to feel that they have become useless and have no control. They also start to believe that they are falling mentally ill.

Dealing With Unpredictable Symptoms

Perimenopause is not only marked by irregular periods but also an array of symptoms that can be unpredictable and difficult to manage. These symptoms originate from the complicated interplay of hormonal changes in the body, mainly involving progesterone and estrogen. The unpredictability and variability of these symptoms make it tough to manage your daily life. Understanding these symptoms will not make this phase disappear or change; however, it will make it easier for you to deal with this phase effectively. Moreover, it can help you feel more informed and less alone as you navigate this complex period in your life.

The unpredictability of these symptoms can change greatly from one person to another; therefore, it is difficult to generalize the experience of perimenopause. For example, some women can have mild symptoms that may occur sporadically, while others can face severe symptoms that largely disrupt their everyday lives.

Below, we will discuss some of the most common symptoms.

One of the common and disruptive symptoms of perimenopause is absolutely the occurrence of hot flashes and night sweats. When these episodes occur anytime and without any warning and last up to several minutes, women start to feel frustrated for many reasons, like:

1. They cannot control it.

2. They cannot ignore it.

3. Their sleep gets disturbed, and sometimes they cannot even get back to sleep.

4. They feel daytime fatigue.

5. They cannot function properly during the day as they are tired and exhausted.

6. If these episodes turn extreme, they feel miserable.

Irregular menstrual cycles are also a hallmark of perimenopause. Due to varying hormone levels, periods do not remain normal at all -with changes in duration, frequency, and flow. Some women may experience menorrhagia, while others might have to deal with oligomenorrhea. This irregularity can be both inconvenient and frustrating, impacting everything from personal life and routine to emotional well-being.

In addition to these symptoms, many women may observe changes in their hair and skin. Decreasing levels of estrogen can lead to diminished production of collagen that results in in drier and less elastic skin. Wrinkles become more pronounced. Hair may also become more brittle and thinner. Although these changes are totally a part of the natural aging cycle, they can be distressing at times as they make you feel that nothing is in your control anymore ranging from your appearance to your daily life activities (Thornton, 2013).

Cognitive symptoms, also referred to as "brain fog," are also part of perimenopause. These can include challenges with concentration, memory lapses, and a constant general feeling of mental cloudiness. These cognitive changes are thought to be associated with hormonal fluctuations and can interfere with your daily chores, activities, and professional responsibilities, adding another thick layer of unpredictability to the experience of perimenopause (Greendale et al., 2011).

The key driver of cognitive symptoms during perimenopause is the instability in hormone levels, particularly progesterone and estrogen. Estrogen plays a vital role in cognitive function by supporting neurotransmitter systems, such as acetylcholine, which is required for learning and memory. As levels of estrogen fluctuate and eventually decrease, the efficiency of the neurotransmitter systems can be compromised, contributing to cognitive difficulties (Greendale et al., 2011).

The irregular sleep patterns also make it hard to maintain a consistent and restorative sleep schedule.

Additionally, vaginal and urinary changes are other symptoms that can appear unpredictably during perimenopause. Lowered estrogen levels cause vaginal atrophy, which further invites itching, dryness, and discomfort during intercourse. Some women can experience urinary incontinence or enhanced frequency of urination. These symptoms can be random and embarrassing, further contributing to the sense of loss of control and unpredictability.

Weight gain and other changes in body composition are very common and unpredictable. But when this shift occurs in body composition when some women are already trying to maintain regular exercise and healthy eating habits, they feel frustrated, upset, and depressed.

Grieving the Loss of Reproductive Ability

The transition through perimenopause indicates the end of a woman's reproductive years, a very significant milestone that can give birth to complex emotions. For example, that phase can bring forth a sense of grief as women have to come to terms with the end of their fertility.

Consider the example of Amanda in her mid-40s who wishes to and has been trying to conceive her second child for many years. As she enters the perimenopausal period and comes to know that her chances of conceiving are at stake, she experiences a deep sense of loss and grief. Her dreams of growing her family and giving her only child a sibling are now unlikely to be fulfilled, signaling a period of adjustment and mourning. So, she has to deal with this grief.

Emotional Impact

The loss of reproductive ability can trigger a deep emotional response in many women. For many women, fertility is closely linked with their identity and life plans. The actualization that they can no longer conceive children can lead to feelings of loss, sadness, and even mourning, similar to the suffering and grief experienced with other major life changes. This emotional response is not merely about the physical capability to conceive but also about the expectations, dreams, and social roles tied to fertility.

Women who had hoped to have more children or have been trying to conceive can feel this loss more acutely. The end of the reproductive cycle can symbolize the end of those aspirations and dreams, leading to a profound sense of unfulfilled desire and regret. Even women who do not have any plans to have more children can undergo this feeling due to the cultural and societal significance placed both on fertility and motherhood.

Biological and Social Factors

Biologically, the cessation of reproductive power is quite a natural part of aging. As women age, the number along with the quality of their oocytes (egg cells) declines, and the fertility rate also decreases. This process is slow and typically starts in a woman's mid-to-late 30s, accelerating in her 40s. By the time a woman arrives at perimenopause, her ovarian reserve—the collection of available eggs—is extremely diminished, marking the conclusion of her natural reproductive ability(Secomandi et al., 2021).

Socially, motherhood and fertility are often celebrated and valued parts of a woman's life. Society places great emphasis on the ability of a woman to bear children, and they unconsciously feel pressure to conform to these expectations.

The end can thus also be seen as a loss of societal status and value, leading to feelings of diminished self-worth and inadequacy. This societal pressure can heighten the grief experienced during this transition.

Personal Narratives and Identity

The loss of reproductive potential can also impact a woman's narrative and personal sense of identity. Many women recognize strongly their role as either mothers or potential mothers. The end of this period can result in an identity crisis, as women now need to reframe their self-concept and find new ways to define their value and purpose. This approach can be emotionally taxing and challenging, especially for those who have placed great importance on their fertility.

For other women, the loss of reproductive ability can bring about an enhanced sense of relief and liberation. They may feel free from the biological and societal pressures of fertility and be able to explore new parts of their identity and life goals. However, this positive perspective can not negate the complex emotions and grief that usually accompany the transition.

Impact on Mental Health

We have already discussed that hormonal changes enhance the risk of developing mental health issues, such as depression and anxiety disorders during perimenopause. Let's discuss them in more detail.

Biological Factors

The hormonal changes during perimenopause can largely enhance the risk of anxiety and depression. Estrogen and progesterone regulate the menstrual cycle and play important roles in mood regulation and brain function. As their levels keep on changing, they can disrupt the balance of neurotransmitters, like serotonin and dopamine, that maintain mood stability. The decrease in estrogen, in particular, has been tied to reduced serotonin levels, which can give birth to mood disorders.

Psychological Stress

The psychological stress during perimenopause can heighten the risk of getting depression and anxiety. Many women face increased life stressors during this period, such as experiencing changes in their family dynamics (children leaving home), caring for aging parents, and navigating professional pressures. The collective effect of these stressors blended with the physical symptoms of perimenopause (like sleep disturbances and hot flashes), can build a fertile ground for mental health challenges to emerge.

According to a study, women in perimenopause are twice as likely to experience depressive symptoms compared to premenopausal ones (Women Are 40% More Likely to Experience Depression during the Perimenopause, 2024). Another study emphasized that perimenopausal women are at higher risk for developing anxiety, highlighting the need for awareness and proper mental health care during this transitional period (Alblooshi et al., 2023).

Increased Vulnerability

Women who have a history of anxiety or depression are particularly vulnerable to experiencing these symptoms during perimenopause. Studies have revealed that women with a prior history of mood conditions are more likely to experience a recurrence during this period (Alblooshi et al., 2023). Additionally, those who have encountered premenstrual dysphoric disorder (PMDD) or postpartum depression are at a heightened risk, suggesting that sensitivity to hormonal changes plays an important role (Lee et al., 2015).

Symptoms and Diagnosis

The symptoms of depression and anxiety can be very similar to those experienced at other times but may be aggravated by concurrent physical symptoms. Common symptoms of depression are:

- persistent sadness
- loss of interest in daily activities and important tasks

- changes in weight

- changes in appetite

- sleep disturbances

- feelings of guilt or worthlessness

Anxiety symptoms can entail:

- excessive worry

- restlessness

- anger

- irritability

- muscle tension

- difficulty concentrating

Diagnosing depression and anxiety at this stage can be very difficult due to the overlap of psychological and physical symptoms. Healthcare providers need to consider the context of hormonal variations and the presence of perimenopausal symptoms when evaluating mental health. Comprehensive assessments that include psychological assessment, medical history, and consideration of hormonal status are required for a proper and accurate diagnosis.

The impact of anxiety and depression on everyday life can be profound. You may find it difficult to perform common tasks, maintain relationships and professional contacts, and fulfill professional responsibilities. The cognitive symptoms tied to perimenopause, such as memory lapses and difficulty concentrating, can be worsened by anxiety and depression, leading to a decline in overall functioning.

Feeling Overwhelmed and Unable to Cope

When your body and mind are going through so many changes, dealing with them can seem very overwhelming. These changes can often leave you feeling unable to cope with even daily demands. That is a totally natural feeling; therefore, you must understand all about this universal phase of life.

Hormonal fluctuations are a basic part of perimenopause. The irregular levels can directly influence your emotional stability and mood. This hormonal volatility makes it difficult for you to maintain your emotional equilibrium. As a result, you start to feel overwhelmed.

Likewise, the physical condition of perimenopause can be disruptive and exhausting, further leading to the enhanced sense of being overwhelmed. Hot flashes, sleep disturbances, and night sweats can lead to persistent sleep deprivation. This lack of quality sleep, in turn, impairs cognitive function, diminishes patience, and minimizes overall resilience, making it harder to handle everyday stressors.

Fatigue is a common symptom that can largely sap your energy levels, leaving you with little reserve for managing your usual activities. The cumulative effect of these physical symptoms can sometimes take the form of constant struggle, where even little tasks feel insurmountable.

The psychological and emotional stress is another main factor. Many women face many concurrent stressors during this period, such as experiencing changes in personal relationships. These stressors can compound the emotional effect of hormonal changes, cultivating consistent heightened feelings of being overwhelmed.

Additionally, societal expectations and pressures about aging and productivity can make these feelings unbearable. Women can feel pressured to retain their roles and responsibilities in spite of the emotional and physical challenges they are experiencing. This pressure can lead to a sense of failure and inadequacy when they are unable to meet these expectations.

Cognitive symptoms can contribute to the feeling of being overwhelmed. Known as brain fog, these symptoms can make it very difficult for you to focus on tasks, memorize important information, and make informed decisions. This cognitive impairment can also lead to frustration and a lower sense of competency, further adding to the stress of managing your daily life.

The family and social dynamics that usually accompany perimenopause can also play a part. Some women in this stage of life are balancing multiple roles, ranging from being a partner and caregiver to a parent and being a professional. The needs of these roles can be overwhelming, especially when followed by the physical and emotional challenges of perimenopause. For instance, a woman who is caring for her aging parents while managing a household and career at the same time may find herself in trouble. The competing demands on her energy and time can lead to burnout and feelings of not trying or giving enough. This condition is further complicated by the societal expectation that a woman should always be able to handle all the roles seamlessly.

Another example is when children are leaving home. The empty nest syndrome can result in a profound sense of change and loss in family dynamics. Women who have devoted a large portion of their energy and time to raising their children may find it strangely difficult to adjust to their absence (Bougea et al., 2020). This change can leave a void and invite feelings of purposelessness that overwhelm them as they need to redefine their roles and find new activities to fill their time.

Changes in personal relationships can also become a source of stress. Perimenopause can coincide with a time when long-term relationships, like marriages, may undergo substantial transformations. Some couples may face enhanced marital strain due to the stress of perimenopause and changing life circumstances. This strain can make them feel isolated and emotionally overwhelmed.

Importance of Emotional Support

This transitional period undoubtedly brings with it a myriad of emotional, physical, and psychological challenges. During this time, the significance and need for emotional support cannot be overlooked. When nothing is working, some words and kind gestures accompanied by the realization that "I am here for you" can make a large difference.

Having a strong support system can affect how women cope with the transitions and challenges in this phase. Emotional support from friends, family, and healthcare professionals can offer the understanding, reassurance, and comfort essential for navigating perimenopause more effectively.

Emotional Stability and Mental Health

One of the key benefits of emotional support during perimenopause is the rise of emotional stability for mental health. Hormonal fluctuations can contribute to anxiety, mood swings, and depression and women cannot maintain a positive outlook easily. Emotional support will act as a buffer against these negative and unhealthy feelings for them. When women have someone to confide in, share their experiences with, and receive encouragement and appreciation from, they are more likely to feel less isolated and misunderstood. This sense of connection can release feelings of depression and anxiety, contributing to overall mental health and well-being.

For example, when you are talking to a close friend about the frustrations of your sleep disturbances or hot flashes it can offer you a sense of validation and relief. Knowing that someone is there who not only understands but also acknowledges your struggles can make these challenges feel more manageable and less overwhelming.

Strengthening Relationships

Emotional support is also very important for strengthening relationships. The changes that occur during perimenopause can strain relationships with partners, family members, and friends. Open communication and mutual support can help maintain and even strengthen these bonds. When partners and family members are supportive and understanding, it can lead to a more harmonious home environment, reducing stress and conflict.

For example, a partner who listens and offers empathy when a woman is experiencing mood swings or physical discomfort can help her feel more supported and less alone. This understanding can enhance the emotional connection between partners and foster a sense of teamwork in navigating the challenges of perimenopause together.

Validation and Normalization of Experiences

Emotional support provides validation and normalization of experiences. Many women may feel ashamed or embarrassed by the symptoms they experience during perimenopause, such as weight gain, changes in libido, or hot flashes. Emotional support from others who have experienced the same or even who are knowledgeable about this phase can help normalize these signs and lower feelings of shame.

Support groups, whether online or in-person, can be particularly helpful in this regard. Sharing stories as well as hearing about others' experiences can comfort women that what they are going through is very normal and that they are not alone in this journey. This validation can also minimize feelings of loneliness and increase self-esteem.

According to the research, women who have higher levels of social support had decreased levels of anxiety and depressive symptoms during perimenopause (Alblooshi et al., 2023).

Encouragement and Motivation

Having a robust support system can also give you motivation and encouragement. Navigating the physical and emotional symptoms of perimenopause can be very taxing, and women can sometimes feel like giving up on goals or activities they once enjoyed. Supportive family and friends can provide the encouragement needed to pursue hobbies, stay active, and maintain social connections effectively.

For example, a partner who encourages you to continue your regular exercise routine despite weariness can help you maintain physical well-being and emotional health. Exercise has been revealed to alleviate some symptoms of perimenopause, such as sleep disturbances and mood swings, and having a workout buddy in the form of your partner can make it easier to stay motivated and happy (Qian et al., 2023).

A recent study reveals that emotional support from partners significantly enhances a woman's coping strategies and helps her maintain overall mental health during this period (Qian et al., 2023).

Access to Resources and Information

Emotional support also comes hand in hand with access to information and resources. Family, friends, and support groups can give you valuable insights into managing symptoms, exploring effective treatments, and accessing healthcare services. This collective knowledge can empower and help women to make informed decisions about their overall health and well-being.

For instance, a support group member can recommend a healthcare professional who specializes in perimenopausal care or share useful information about dietary supplements that have helped them with their symptoms. This type of practical support can improve a woman's skills to cope with perimenopause and enhance her quality of life.

As we understand the emotional transformations of perimenopause, it is equally significant to address the social challenges that also accompany this stage of life. In the next chapter, we will mainly focus on social challenges.

Chapter 3: Social Challenges

There is no greater agony than bearing an untold story inside you. -Maya Angelou

As women navigate the physical and emotional transitions of perimenopause, they often encounter a wide range of social challenges that can complicate this already challenging period. In this chapter, we will understand these social dynamics as they are important for managing the broader effects of perimenopause on a woman's life.

Interpersonal Relationships

Interpersonal relationships during perimenopause can be greatly affected by the physical and emotional variations that women experience.

Partner Relationships

One important impact is on marital or long-term partnerships. Studies have suggested that the irritability, mood swings, and anxiety tied to perimenopause can strain even the most solid relationships (Bromberger & Kravitz, 2011). For example, a study highlighted that many women reported an enhanced rate of conflicts with their partners during perimenopause (Sexton, 2022).

Partners find it difficult to understand the quick changes in mood and behavior that lead to tension and miscommunication. The unpredictable nature of these emotional challenges can also lead to frustrations and misunderstandings as partners struggle to empathize with the experiences of their partners undergoing perimenopause.

Furthermore, sexual relationships can be impacted. Vaginal dryness and a lowered libido, common during this phase can create both discomfort and distance between partners.

For instance, when a woman is less inclined to engage in sexual activity, it can create feelings of confusion or rejection for her partner. Sometimes, women show anger toward their spouses without any obvious reason (Sexton, 2022). That is why both partners need to understand that these changes are a normal part of perimenopause.

Social and Workplace Relationships

Besides this, social relationships can be affected to a large extent. Women may find it easy to withdraw themselves from social activities due to symptoms, like hot flashes and fatigue. Feelings of isolation and loneliness can come to the surface due to these withdrawals. For example, a woman can feel that her frequent need to excuse herself to manage sudden episodes of hot flashes makes her feel embarrassed and less willing to attend social gatherings. Consequently, her friends can misinterpret this withdrawal as a lack of commitment or interest, further straining friendships.

Workplace relationships are also influenced by perimenopause. Conditions like cognitive changes or brain fog can impact a woman's work performance and interactions with colleagues. Cognitive decline in the form of memory lapses and lack of concentration can result in mistakes and missed deadlines, which may be misinterpreted by both coworkers and supervisors as a lack of interest or incompetence. Moreover, workplace tensions start to take place and even impact a woman's career advancement opportunities.

Family Dynamics

In family dynamics, the influence of perimenopause is multifaceted. For women as mothers, the symptoms of perimenopause can overlap with the challenges of raising adolescents, building a potentially volatile home atmosphere. Research indicates that perimenopausal women experience elevated tension with teenage children, often because both parties experience major hormonal changes simultaneously. In addition to this, the emotional volatility and exhaustion associated with perimenopause can lower a woman's patience level and the energy required for parenting, leading to more recurring conflicts and an enhanced sense of guilt over perceived inadequacies.

On a positive note, some women also find that discussing their experiences with supportive family members or friends can deepen their bonds. Mutual understanding and empathy can help them enjoy deeper connections and a sense of solidarity. For example, a group of women can form a support network, sharing experiences and tips, which can offer emotional comfort and a sense of fellowship.

Comprehending the technical aspects of perimenopause, including the role of gonadotropin-releasing hormone (GnRH) and the reduction in ovarian follicle activity, can also be helpful in fostering empathy and support from those around the woman experiencing these variations.

Just like estrogen and progesterone, GnRH is also a hormone that is produced by the hypothalamus in the brain and stimulates the pituitary gland to release luteinizing hormone (LH) and follicle-stimulating hormone (FSH). These hormones further regulate the function of the ovaries. During perimenopause, the receptive ability of ovarian follicles to LH and FSH diminishes which also creates a decline in progesterone and estrogen production. This reduction in ovarian follicle activity is a main factor in the symptoms appearing during perimenopause (Marques et al., 2018).

Let us understand this with the help of an example. When ovarian follicles become less active or less responsive, the regularity of menstrual cycles starts to diminish, and ovulation becomes quite unpredictable. This also results in irregular periods and symptoms, like night sweats and hot flashes. The reduced ovarian response also leads to changes in cognition and mood experienced during this time.

Professional Life

As we have already discussed perimenopause can largely impact a woman's professional life, affecting her job satisfaction, performance, and workplace relationships. Fatigue, mood swings, and difficulty concentrating can minimize productivity and enhance absenteeism. For example, if you are experiencing severe hot flashes, you may find it very hard to concentrate during presentations or meetings. It affects your confidence and perceived competence. Also, the stigma surrounding perimenopause can create a lack of understanding and support from your colleagues and managers. This turns your work environment into a challenging environment where you may feel undervalued, unappreciated, or isolated. Identifying and addressing these professional issues is important for fostering an inclusive and supportive workplace.

Challenges in the Workplace

The challenges you may face in the workplace during perimenopause are multi-layered and can include:

Cognitive and Physical Symptoms

Memory lapses, difficulty focusing, or brain fog can impair your job performance. Some women cannot bring themselves to focus on tasks, remember important details, or make quick and good decisions, which are very important in a professional setting. Physical symptoms, such as hot flashes, the constant urge to eat, and exhaustion, on the other hand, can lead to reduced productivity as well as frequent absences.

For example, a woman who experiences severe night sweats will come to work exhausted and tired. It will affect her ability to focus and perform effectively. What will be the consequence? This can result in missed deadlines and poor job performance, which will be misunderstood by employers as either a lack of professionalism or commitment.

Workplace Environment

The workplace atmosphere can aggravate the challenges of perimenopause. Lack of temperature control, unsupportive policies, and inadequate rest facilities can make it hard for most women to manage their symptoms effectively. Similarly, the stigma tied to perimenopause signifies that women may feel very uncomfortable discussing their symptoms with colleagues or managers which also leads to a lack of necessary accommodations.

For example, an open-plan office without enough ventilation will definitely make it tough for a woman experiencing hot flashes to find some moments of relief, increasing her stress levels and discomfort.

Discrimination and Bias

There is primarily a lack of understanding and awareness of perimenopause in the workplace, contributing to potential discrimination and bias. Women can face ageism and sexism, being perceived as less committed, professional, or capable due to their changing symptoms. This can also affect their opportunities for professional advancement, promotion, and overall career development.

Moreover, according to the research, most women experiencing perimenopausal symptoms sometimes not only feel marginalized but also face serious negative stereotypes

(Yeager, 2023). This impacts their job satisfaction, mental health, and career progression.

Mental Health Impact

The constant stress of managing perimenopausal symptoms while maintaining professional obligations can take a heavy toll on mental health. Anxiety, restlessness, and depression keep on testing a woman's mind. Meanwhile, the pressure and need to perform well at work can exacerbate these conditions. When they cannot manage these symptoms or do not get proper support from their colleagues or supervisors, the feelings of anger and frustration also multiply, which further impacts their mental well-being. In simple words, it creates a loop that makes their mental condition only worse.

For example, a woman dealing with depression cannot easily engage in workplace interactions or even maintain her usual level of productivity, which can be translated to as disengagement or lack of seriousness.

Considering Career Changes or Early Retirement

When a woman is going through so many emotional, physical, and cognitive challenges during perimenopause, she starts to evaluate every aspect of her life. She may start to think:

- *Am I doing it right?*

- *Can I ever perform well at work?*

- *Why does everything seem so difficult to handle?*

- *I cannot manage multiple things right now. Maybe it is time I should let go of some things.*

When these thoughts keep on lingering, some women feel it necessary to consider early retirement or career changes. The collective stress of managing signs while trying to maintain professional responsibilities often triggers a reevaluation of career plans and work-life balance.

Physical and Cognitive Demands

During perimenopause, women experience physical and cognitive demands that affect their capability to perform their jobs effectively. Brain fog can hinder their everyday functioning and minimize productivity. For instance, a woman who is working in a high-stress and physically challenging job may find it very difficult to keep up with the pace due to extreme fatigue and reduced stamina. Likewise, a surgeon experiencing constant hot flashes or tremors can notice that her energy and skill to perform her job safely and effectively is compromised, making her reconsider a less demanding position or even early retirement.

Emotional and Psychological Impact

The emotional toll of perimenopause can also force career changes. Persistent mood swings, irritability, and persistent anxiety blur the judgment of women, which can easily impact workplace relationships and overall job contentment. Some women can feel very overwhelmed by the dual demands of overcoming their symptoms and fulfilling professional roles. For instance, if you are experiencing intense mood swings most of the time, you can struggle to maintain your professional demeanor. Sometimes you can find yourself stranded in conflicts with your colleagues or supervisors. Other times, you feel that you should not be doing anything as you are not good enough. So, you are only wasting your time. Meanwhile, the stress of balancing your health and work can prompt a wish for a less stressful or more flexible job.

Workplace Environment

It is true that a workplace environment plays a huge role in a woman's decision to reconsider her career and goals. A stressful, toxic, or unsupportive work setting can worsen perimenopausal symptoms and lead to enhanced job dissatisfaction. A woman, for example, who is working in a highly competitive corporate atmosphere can find the pressure to perform extraordinary and the lack of understanding from her supervisors very intolerable. This could compel her to look for a different role or leave the current workforce entirely.

On the contrary, a supportive work environment that always accommodates the needs of perimenopausal women can help a woman in managing these challenges. A study says that workplace accommodations can significantly minimize the possibility of women leaving the workforce prematurely (O'Neill et al., 2023). Flexible work hours, the availability to work from home, and a culture of awareness and understanding can make it easier for her to mitigate her symptoms while remaining productive and present. However, there are few workplaces that offer such accommodations, which can easily influence the decision to change careers or retire at such an early age.

Reevaluating Priorities

Perimenopause also coincides with other major life transitions, such as elder children leaving home, a partner getting distant, or the need to care for parents. These changes can force women to reevaluate their priorities immediately and consider whether their current ideal career aligns with their long-term dreams and well-being. For instance, a woman who has given decades to a demanding profession may decide that it is time to do part-time work, pursue a passion project, or simply a job that offers a better work-life balance.

Financial Considerations

When women are considering early retirement, they are also assessing financial readiness as well. So, when you are considering leaving your job, you need to evaluate whether you have enough savings, retirement funds, and health insurance to support yourself without a steady income. Financial planning is very crucial as early retirement can affect pension benefits as well as future financial security.

A woman considering early retirement at the age of 55 will need to look at many years without income before she can have access to pension benefits or Social Security. She may need to factor in the cost of potential medical expenses and health insurance given the enhanced likelihood of health issues as she ages. Such financial considerations can impact the decision to retire early are multifaceted and complex.

Societal Attitudes Towards Aging and Perimenopause

Societal attitudes toward perimenopause and aging largely influence women's experiences during this phase. These attitudes impact how women see themselves, how they are treated by others, and how much support they receive.

Understanding these societal dynamics can foster a more supportive and empathetic environment for women undergoing this change.

Ageism and Gender Stereotypes

Ageism or prejudice against older people merged with gender stereotypes, can negatively affect women experiencing perimenopause. Society usually values beauty and youth, leading to the marginalization of older men and women. This can result in feeling invisible and having low self-worth. For example, a woman in her 50s can feel pressured to maintain a youthful appearance and conceal signs of aging under make-up or a fake smile to remain relevant in her social and professional circles. These societal pressures, in reality, can only exacerbate the emotional dilemmas of perimenopause, making it harder for women to deal with their symptoms and maintain a positive self-image.

Lack of Awareness and Understanding

There are often times a lack of awareness and knowledge about perimenopause and its outcomes. Many people, including family members and employers, may not identify the importance of perimenopausal symptoms, contributing to a lack of support. This ignorance can cause dismissive attitudes, where symptoms are either misunderstood or trivialized. For example, a woman can be labeled as "difficult," "too sensitive," or "moody" by her colleagues who are unaware of the hormonal fluctuations that are affecting her mood and behavior. This lack of basic knowledge can create an unsupportive and hostile environment, both at home and at work, further adding to the stress and emotional toll of this stage.

Cultural Norms and Expectations

Cultural norms and expectations about perimenopause and aging vary widely, impacting how women experience this change. In many cultures, perimenopause is seen positively, as a time of gaining more wisdom and freedom. In others, it is stigmatized and looked down upon, and women may feel afraid, embarrassed, or ashamed about their current condition. For example, in many Western societies, where productivity and youth are highly appreciated and valued, women can feel a sense of inadequacy or loss during perimenopause (Grandey et al., 2019). On the other hand, in some Indigenous cultures, elder women are respected, and their menopausal transition is seen as a normal, natural, and respected stage of life. These cultural differences emphasize the significance of societal context in shaping a woman's experiences and attitudes toward perimenopause.

Media Representation

Media representation of aging and perimenopause cannot be overstated in shaping societal attitudes. Positive and realistic descriptions can help normalize the changes in perimenopausal women and minimize stigma. However, inaccurate or negative portrayals can perpetuate stereotypes and myths, leading to prejudice and misunderstandings. For example, media depicting perimenopausal women as overly emotional or irrational reinforces negative stereotypes and can impact public perception. A media that underscores the achievements and powers of older women, on the contrary, can help shift societal attitudes toward a more supportive view of perimenopause and aging.

According to Cowell et al., positive and supportive cultural attitudes toward perimenopause are closely associated with better coping strategies as well as overall well-being (2024).

Internalized Ageism and Shame

Internalized ageism and shame can deeply influence women during perimenopause. These internalized feelings and beliefs can largely influence a woman's emotional and psychological challenges during this transition, leading to a diminished sense of self-worth and elevated levels of stress.

Understanding Internalized Ageism

In the words of Frances McDormand, "Ageism is a cultural illness; it's not a personal illness" (Applewhite, 2014).

Internalized ageism involves the acceptance as well as internalization of negative attitudes and stereotypes about aging by the people who are the targets of these stereotypes. When society regularly devalues aging, older men and women may start to believe these societal messages leading to self-stigmatization. Particularly for women experiencing the changes during perimenopause, this can manifest in several ways, including decreased self-esteem, feelings of inadequacy, and shame about their changing capabilities and bodies.

For instance, a woman who has internalized ageist beliefs can see her perimenopausal symptoms, such as wrinkles or weight gain, as signs of unattractiveness or failure, even the fact that they are only natural occurrences. This internalized ageism can contribute to negative self-talk, where she will criticize herself for not preserving a youthful appearance or for undergoing cognitive changes, like memory lapses.

The signs of internal ageism can be:

- You do not want to be associated with older people in any way.

- You obsess about having a youthful and cheerful appearance and try to look young.

- You feel as if you have nothing to give to the world just because of your age (Schoenwald, 2024). In other words, you have become useless in your personal and professional life.

What Women See Affects Them

Media and cultural norms have a lion's share in the development of internalized ageism. Advertising, television, and movies often glorify youth and portray aging in negative colors. Older women are regularly depicted as unattractive, useless, burdensome, or irrelevant, while youth is linked with vitality, success, and beauty. These pervasive media messages strengthen societal values that prioritize almost everything over age, resulting in the internalization of ageist attitudes by women.

Moreover, anti-aging products are advertised aggressively, promoting the idea that aging is something a woman is supposed to be fighting against instead of embracing. When women are exposed to these messages, they feel forced to invest in expensive treatments and cosmetics in order to maintain a youthful appearance, hiding their sense of shame about their natural aging process.

Shame and Its Impact

Shame is a very powerful and sometimes debilitating emotion that can emerge from internalized ageism. It entails feeling deeply unworthy or flawed due to your *perceived* shortcomings. For perimenopausal women, shame arises from their physical changes, diminished fertility, or perceived loss of competence and desirability.

This shame can further impact several aspects of a woman's life. In a social environment, she may prefer to withdraw or avoid tasks where her age might be discussed or noticed. At work, she may feel less capable and confident than others, particularly if she is experiencing symptoms, like brain fog or fatigue. This lack of confidence can also lead to self-sabotage, such as not sharing ideas in meetings or avoiding taking on new duties, which in turn can influence career progression and job satisfaction.

Importance of Raising Awareness and Promoting Understanding

In a small town, there lived a woman named Mary who had always prided herself on her lively spirit and youthful exuberance. When she approached her late 50s, Mary started to observe subtle changes in her mind and body that made her feel less confident and inadequate. Her once sharp memory started to vanish away, and she experienced recurring bouts of fatigue. In spite of these natural transitions, she found herself struggling with a deep-seated feeling of inadequacy (Harvey A. Friedman Center for Aging, 2023).

This feeling of inadequacy was not merely about the physical changes she was undergoing; it was also stemming from societal attitudes toward aging. Mary's internalized ageism made her realize that her value was decreasing with every passing year. She was frequently bombarded by societal messages and media that correlated youth with value and vitality with success. These messages started to seep into her own self-perception, making her view aging as a personal failing instead of a natural life stage (Harvey A. Friedman Center for Aging, 2023).

One day, Mary saw an article that discussed internalized ageism and its influence. It was nothing less than a revelation. It explained to her that many people unknowingly adopt society's negative stereotypes and thinking about aging which leads to self-discrimination and diminished self-worth. She also realized that her sense of inadequacy was not unique but a very common experience imposed by societal norms.

Inspired by this newfound piece of knowledge, Mary started to challenge these internalized beliefs. She joined a community group where members shared their experiences and supported one another in embracing aging positively and open-mindedly. With time, Mary learned to appreciate her own unique experiences and wisdom instead of solely focusing on her physical appearance. She embraced the fact that her value wasn't dependent upon her age but on her attitudes and actions (Harvey A. Friedman Center for Aging, 2023).

Mary is not the only woman whose awareness made her experience more relaxing. You can also enjoy this process. All you need is the power of awareness and understanding.

Raising awareness as well as promoting understanding about perimenopause and its associated challenges will also help you improve the lives of women undergoing this phase. By addressing the gaps in knowledge and building a supportive setting, society can greatly impact the emotional, physical, and social well-being of women.

Bridging Knowledge Gaps

One of the main reasons for raising awareness is to bridge the knowledge gaps encircling perimenopause. Despite its universality and prevalence of challenges, many people lack a deep understanding of the symptoms along with the implications of this life phase. Even 90% of women have never been told anything about perimenopause in their schools (Harper et al., 2022). This lack of knowledge can contribute to stigmatization and misconceptions, which worsen the challenges women face. For instance, without enough education, people can misinterpret symptoms, like sleep disturbances or mood swings as simply signs of stress or personal failings, instead of identifying them as legitimate parts of perimenopause.

Educational initiatives, like public health campaigns and informational resources, play the main role in dispelling myths and stereotypes and offering accurate information. By informing both the healthcare professionals and the general public, these initiatives can ensure that women get the support and understanding they need and deserve. For example, educational programs in communities and workplaces can help lower stigma and foster a more empathetic approach to women during perimenopause. They can state that women in this stage experience different symptoms, with 68.9% of mood swings 68.3% of brain fog, and 66.8% of fatigue (Harper et al., 2022).

Fostering Empathy and Support

Promoting awareness about perimenopause also cultivates empathy and support from friends, family, and colleagues. When people are informed about the issues related to perimenopause, they are more likely to provide practical support and emotional encouragement. As Brené Brown writes, "Empathy is the key that unlocks the door to understanding and connection" (The Blinkist Team, 2023). This can affect a woman's ability to cope with symptoms and adopt a positive outlook.

Moreover, a study found that women who get support from their social networks reported enhanced mental health instances and a more positive experience of perimenopause (Cowell et al., 2024). Contrarily, a lack of understanding and support can result in feelings of frustration and isolation. By raising awareness, we all can build an environment where women feel supported and validated, rather than misunderstood or marginalized.

Improving Healthcare and Workplace Environments

Awareness and understanding are equally essential for enhancing healthcare and workplace environments. In healthcare, comprehensive knowledge about perimenopause can contribute to more accurate diagnoses and customized treatment plans. Healthcare officials who are well-informed about the different symptoms and effects of perimenopause are better prepared to give appropriate care and interventions.

In the workplace, comprehending perimenopause can result in creating more supportive policies and practices. For example, flexible work arrangements along with wellness programs that acknowledge the issues and demands of perimenopause can enhance job performance and satisfaction.

Addressing Societal Attitudes and Stereotypes

Raising awareness also encompasses addressing common stereotypes and societal attitudes associated with aging and perimenopause. Unhealthy stereotypes and cultural taboos can internalize stigma and impede open discussions about perimenopause. For example, media portrayals regularly depict perimenopause as a negative experience, supporting stereotypes about aging and decreasing the perceived value of older women. By promoting accurate and positive representations, we can challenge these stereotypes effectively and foster a more supportive and inclusive society.

Campaigns and advocacy efforts that stress the positive aspects of aging and the contributions of older women can help change societal attitudes. For example, initiatives that celebrate the accomplishments and wisdom of older women can counteract toxic stereotypes and promote a more positive view of aging.

Enhancing Research and Policy Development

Comprehensive awareness can also drive advancements in research and policy development. When the public and policymakers know about the challenges of perimenopause, there is a greater impetus to invest in the field of research and craft policies that address these challenges. Research funding as well as policy initiatives that emphasize enriching the quality of life for women during perimenopause can lead to better treatments as well as support systems.

For example, research that explores the consequences of perimenopause on different aspects of life, such as workplace performance, mental health, and social relationships, can offer valuable insights for creating targeted interventions. Also, policy changes that address healthcare coverage as well as workplace accommodations can greatly improve the experiences of women.

Once you have gained enough knowledge of social changes, the final step is to seek help. In the following chapter, we will learn about how to seek help and find effective solutions.

Chapter 4: Seeking Help and Finding Solutions

All problems become smaller when you confront them instead of dodging them. -William F. Halsey

Once you have understood the transitional phase of perimenopause, you have already dealt with half of the problem. The next step is to get in touch with a healthcare professional who can not only clear your doubts but also give you directions on what to do next. Based on your condition, they can suggest you go for Hormonal Replacement Therapy or change your lifestyle. In this chapter, we will look into different possible solutions that can help you manage symptoms of perimenopause.

Why Should A Woman Seek Help?

There is often stigma and shame associated with seeking help for your mental well-being. But don't you think that is totally absurd and unfair?

As you take care of your physical health, you should also book an appointment with a healthcare professional when you feel that you are unable to enjoy sound mental and emotional health. Everyone needs to adopt this attitude toward mental and emotional health. There is no doubt that mental health is as important as physical health and maybe more than physical health as your mental health can affect your physical health.

Seeking help during tough times, such as those experienced during the transitional phase of perimenopause or other major life changes, can help you maintain both mental and physical well-being. There are many other compelling reasons why reaching out for help can be useful.

Professional Expertise

Healthcare providers, including therapists, doctors, and counselors, offer in-depth knowledge and expertise that can prove invaluable. They can understand your specific needs. For example, a therapist with knowledge of managing mood disorders can give insights and strategies that you can directly apply to your emotional challenges.

Moreover, professionals can address multi-faceted symptoms and co-occurring conditions. For instance, if you're experiencing extreme anxiety or mood swings, a mental health professional can help you differentiate between symptoms associated with hormonal changes and other psychological conditions, ensuring you receive the right and appropriate care.

Emotional and Psychological Benefits

Seeking help gives you an opportunity to be heard, understood, and validated. Talking to a trained counselor or a therapist enables you to share your experiences openly with others who understand exactly what you're going through at this particular moment. This validation can minimize feelings of loneliness and shame and offer reassurance that you are not alone in your journey toward healing.

Mental health professionals can also provide you with strategies for managing emotions and feelings, adopting coping mechanisms, and navigating intricate feelings. Their guidance helps you understand and address psychological stressors, which can contribute to enhanced emotional resilience and overall well-being.

Improved Quality of Life

Seeking help often encompasses a holistic approach that addresses several aspects of health, including emotional, physical, and psychological. For example, a detailed treatment plan for perimenopausal symptoms includes not only a medical cure but also lifestyle modifications, mental health support, and nutritional advice.

Professional support can further enhance daily functioning and life quality. Addressing symptoms such as persistent fatigue with targeted interventions can refine your ability to engage in day-to-day activities, maintain your relationships, and enjoy life more.

Prevention of Complications

Seeking help early can help you prevent symptoms from worsening and also minimize the risk of developing more serious conditions. For example, untreated anxiety or depression can result in significant impairments in functioning, while early intervention can successfully prevent these difficulties and promote a quicker recovery.

Empowerment and Self-Efficacy

By seeking timely help, you gain access to resources and information that empower you to make informed and quick decisions regarding your health. Understanding your options and getting expert advice allows you to actively participate in your care and make constant choices that align with your goals and needs.

Additionally, engaging in support groups or therapy can foster personal self-awareness and growth. Learning more about yourself and your attitude to challenges can increase self-confidence and improve problem-solving skills.

Importance of Open Communication

with Healthcare Providers

Effective communication with providers is important for addressing the multifaceted challenges that occur during perimenopause. Open dialogue ensures accurate diagnosis, and appropriate treatment, and enhances overall support and care throughout this transitional phase.

Ensuring Accurate Diagnosis

One of the key reasons that you should adopt open communication is that it helps you gain accurate diagnosis. Perimenopause is filled with a wide range of symptoms, including mood swings, irregular menstrual cycles, and sleep disturbances, which can sometimes coincide with other medical conditions. For instance, symptoms like anxiety or depression can be attributed to perimenopause, but they can also suggest other underlying issues, such as mental health conditions or thyroid disorders.

By communicating openly with their healthcare officials, women can give a complete picture of their symptoms as well as their health history. This comprehensive information helps healthcare professionals differentiate between perimenopausal symptoms and other potential health situations. For example, a patient experiencing severe mood swings and fatigue may need a thorough assessment to rule out conditions, such as chronic fatigue syndrome or bipolar disorder.

Tailoring Treatment Plans

Effective communication also plays a vital role in creating treatment plans suitable for every different person. Know that perimenopause is not a one-size-fits-all experience; its influence can change significantly from one woman to another. Some women may experience severe symptoms that demand intervention, while others may experience milder symptoms that do not require any medical treatment.

For example, hormone replacement therapy (HRT) can be recommended for some women to deal with symptoms, such as night sweats and hot flashes. However, HRT is not right for everyone, and its use relies upon individual health factors and preferences. By discussing their concerns, symptoms, and treatment goals with their healthcare professionals, women can collaboratively tailor a personalized treatment plan that addresses their specific needs and concerns.

Addressing Concerns and Preferences

Open communication gives women the freedom to express their preferences and concerns regarding treatment options. Some women can have reservations about certain treatments due to personal beliefs or potential side effects. For example, a woman can be hesitant to use hormonal treatments due to anxiety about the risk of cardiovascular issues or breast cancer.

In these cases, healthcare professionals can provide complementary approaches or alternative treatments. For example, if a patient is hesitant to use HRT, her provider can suggest other non-hormonal options, such as selective serotonin reuptake inhibitors (SSRIs) for mood regulation or lifestyle adaptations to manage symptoms. Discussing these preferences honestly helps ensure that the selected treatment aligns with the patient's health goals and values.

Managing Expectations and Education

Managing expectations and offering education about perimenopause becomes easier when you employ honest communication. Understanding what to expect during this stage can help women feel less anxious and more prepared. For instance, knowing that changing hormone levels can cause erratic menstrual cycles and altering symptom intensity can help women better manage their preferences and expectations and minimize frustration.

Healthcare providers can provide valuable information about the natural progression of perimenopause symptoms and available treatment choices. This educational phase is important for empowering women to make informed decisions about their own health and navigate perimenopause with grace and confidence.

Building a Supportive Relationship

A supportive relationship between healthcare providers and patients can address the psychological and emotional aspects of perimenopause. Open communication fosters trust and makes sure that women feel valued and heard. This supportive relationship can make it easier for them to discuss sensitive issues, such as cognitive changes, sexual health, or mental health concerns.

For example, a woman undergoing changes in sexual function or libido can find it tough to discuss these issues with her healthcare professional. However, a non-judgmental and open dialogue can help address these issues and explore appropriate solutions, such as lifestyle adjustments, counseling, or treatment plans.

Monitoring and Adjusting Treatment

Perimenopause is not a static phase, and its symptoms can evolve. Regular communication between patients and healthcare providers enables ongoing monitoring and adjustment of treatment plans when needed. For example, a woman can start with a specific treatment for hot flashes but later discover that her symptoms have changed or new symptoms have appeared.

Regular follow-up appointments as well as open discussions allow healthcare providers to evaluate the effectiveness of the treatment and make adjustments. This continuous feedback loop guarantees that the treatment plan remains responsive and effective to the woman's varying needs.

Navigating Complex Health Issues

Open communication can navigate complex health issues that may emerge during perimenopause. For example, some women can experience that their conditions are becoming more intense day by day, such as hypertension or diabetes, due to changes in metabolism and hormonal shifts. In such circumstances, discussing these issues openly with healthcare professionals can ensure thorough management and coordination of care.

Moreover, they can offer guidance on managing these symptoms in conjunction with perimenopausal symptoms, ensuring that all parts of the woman's health are addressed.

Hormone Replacement Therapy and Other Medical Options

Hormone Replacement Therapy (HRT) and other medical choices are commonly used to manage the symptoms during perimenopause and menopause. Each approach has its own unique benefits, considerations, and risks, which are important for you to understand when exploring different treatment options.

Hormone Replacement Therapy (HRT)

Hormone Replacement Therapy encompasses the administration of hormones to reduce symptoms related to hormonal fluctuations during perimenopause. HRT usually includes progesterone, estrogen, or a combination of both. The combination also depends on whether a woman still has her uterus or has had a hysterectomy (Harper-Harrison & Shanahan, 2023).

Types of HRT

1. **Estrogen-only HRT:** Appropriate for women who have undergone a hysterectomy as they do not require progesterone to protect the uterine lining. This kind of HRT can help relieve symptoms, such as night sweats, vaginal dryness, and hot flashes. Estrogen also helps maintain bone density, minimizing the risk of fractures and osteoporosis.

2. **Combined HRT:** It includes both progesterone and estrogen and is suitable for women who still have their uterus. Progesterone helps prevent the risk of endometrial cancer that can be linked to estrogen alone (Harper-Harrison & Shanahan, 2023).

Risks and Considerations

- **Cardiovascular risks:** Long-term usage of HRT has been linked with an increased risk of heart disease along with stroke.

- **Cancer Risks:** There is an enhanced risk of breast cancer with combined HRT, particularly when it is used for a long time.

- **Side Effects:** Some women can experience side effects, such as headaches, nausea, and mood swings (Harper-Harrison & Shanahan, 2023).

Healthcare providers also consider all these factors when recommending HRT, and treatment plans are usually personalized based on individual health profiles, needs, and preferences.

Non-Hormonal Medical Options

For women who choose not to or cannot use HRT, there are many other non-hormonal medical options available to manage their perimenopausal symptoms:

1. **Selective Serotonin Reuptake Inhibitors (SSRIs):** These medications are commonly used to address depression, but they can also help ease hot flashes and mood swings. SSRIs are often recommended when HRT is not suitable due to personal choice or contraindications (Worth, 2016).

2. **Serotonin-Norepinephrine Reuptake Inhibitors (SNRIs):** Just like SSRIs, SNRIs can also decrease hot flashes and improve mood. They work by enhancing levels of norepinephrine and serotonin in the brain (Cleveland Clinic, 2023).

3. **Gabapentin:** Originally created as an anticonvulsant medication, gabapentin is effective in minimizing hot flashes. It is frequently used when hormonal treatments are not the right fit.

4. **Clonidine:** This medication is used mainly for high blood pressure but can also help with hot flashes. It works by influencing the brain's regulation of body temperature.

5. **Vaginal estrogen:** For localized symptoms, such as discomfort during intercourse and vaginal dryness, vaginal estrogen products (rings, tablets, or creams) deliver estrogen directly to the vaginal region with minimal systemic absorption.

Alternative Therapies

Some women can also explore alternative therapies as part of their management strategy, including:

- **Phytoestrogens:** These are plant-based compounds that mimic estrogen in the body. They are found in foods, such as flaxseeds and soy, and they can offer mild symptom relief (Canivenc-Lavier & Bennetau-Pelissero, 2023).

- **Acupuncture and herbal remedies:** Although some find relief from these approaches, their safety and effectiveness are less well-documented compared to other conventional treatments.

Monitoring and Adjusting Treatment

Regardless of the treatment you choose, you should focus on ongoing monitoring as adjustments are important. Ensure that you have regular follow-ups with your healthcare provider to evaluate the effectiveness of the current treatment and make any necessary adjustments. This can involve adjusting dosages, changing medications, or exploring additional options based on changing symptoms and health conditions.

Lifestyle Modifications

Lifestyle modifications can play a huge difference in managing the symptoms of perimenopause and enhancing overall well-being. These adjustments can help many women alleviate discomfort, improve physical health, and support emotional stability during this transition. Let us have an overview of primary lifestyle changes that can positively affect perimenopausal symptoms.

Diet and Nutrition

Balanced diet: A well-balanced diet rich in vegetables, whole grains, fruits, healthy fats, and lean proteins can help mitigate symptoms, such as mood swings and hot flashes (Erdélyi et al., 2024). Foods rich in phytoestrogens, like flaxseeds, legumes, and soy products, may give mild symptom relief by mimicking estrogen in your body.

Whole grains: Foods like quinoa, oats, and brown rice are high in fiber and can help effectively with digestive health and weight management. Whole grains also offer essential nutrients, like B vitamins as well as magnesium, which support bone health and energy levels.

Lean proteins: Sources, such as fish, chicken, tofu, and legumes are important for maintaining muscle mass as well as overall health. Protein helps manage blood sugar levels and can lead to feeling full, which can help in weight management (Erdélyi et al., 2024).

Calcium and vitamin D: Adequate intake of vitamin D and calcium is important for bone health, particularly as estrogen levels diminish, which can contribute to decreased bone density. Dairy products, leafy green vegetables, fortified plant-based milks, and sunlight exposure can help maintain your bone strength.

Hydration: Staying well-hydrated is also necessary for overall health and can help minimize symptoms, like vaginal dryness and dry skin. Drinking plenty of water throughout the day is very beneficial.

Limit caffeine and alcohol: Lowering caffeine and alcohol consumption can help alleviate symptoms, like sleep disturbances and hot flashes. Both substances can stimulate or exacerbate these symptoms in some women.

Healthy fats: Consider incorporating sources of healthy fats, like nuts, avocados, olive oil, and seeds as they can support cardiovascular health and minimize inflammation. These fats are also beneficial for maintaining skin health and the production of hormones (Erdélyi et al., 2024).

Exercise and Physical Activity

Regular exercise: Engaging in regular physical exercise and activity can largely improve overall health and well-being. Exercise can help improve mood, manage weight, and minimize the risk of cardiovascular disease. Activities, such as brisk walking, swimming, and yoga, are very beneficial (Dhuli et al., 2022).

Strength training: Integrating strength training into your daily routine can help maintain bone density and muscle mass. Resistance exercises, like lifting weights or using resistance bands are very effective in promoting bone health.

Stress reduction: Exercise can also act as a stress reliever, which is vital for managing anxiety and mood swings. Practices, such as yoga and tai chi, not only improve physical fitness but also promote relaxation, emotional, and mental well-being.

Flexibility and balance: Activities, like Pilates and yoga improve balance, flexibility, and overall body strength. These exercises can also relieve stress, enhance sleep quality, and reduce symptoms, such as stiffness and joint pain.

Sleep and Rest

Quality Sleep: Setting a regular sleep routine and building a restful environment can help manage sleep disturbances common during this transitional phase. Maintaining a consistent sleep schedule and setting a calming bedtime routine can enhance sleep quality.

Sleep environment: Optimizing the sleep environment—like keeping the bedroom cool, quiet, and dark—can help manage night sweats and enhance overall sleep quality.

Identify and Avoid Triggers

Keeping a symptom diary to recognize potential triggers for mood swings, hot flashes, or other symptoms can be very helpful. Common triggers can include stress, eating very spicy foods, or certain environmental factors. Once recognized, avoiding these triggers can help you minimize and manage symptom severity.

Stress Management Techniques

Managing stress effectively holds the first position during perimenopause as stress can worsen symptoms, such as hot flashes, mood swings, and sleep disturbances. Implementing several stress management techniques can help enhance overall well-being and maintain a balanced transition through this phase.

You can employ these stress management techniques:

Mindfulness and Meditation

Mindfulness: Practicing mindfulness consists of focusing solely on the present moment and accepting it without judgment or criticism. Techniques, such as mindful breathing, mindfulness meditation, and body scans, can help minimize stress and enhance emotional resilience. Mindfulness practices facilitate awareness of feelings and thoughts, which can help in managing anxiety and depression and improving overall mood.

Meditation: Regular meditation, including transcendental meditation, loving-kindness meditation, or guided meditation, reduces stress and promotes relaxation. Meditative practices can help calm the mind and enhance emotional regulation and focus contributing to an enhanced sense of well-being.

Deep Breathing Exercises

Deep breathing exercises can help activate the body's relaxation response, lowering stress levels and heart rate. Techniques such as paced breathing or diaphragmatic breathing involve taking slow and deep breaths from the diaphragm. It can help calm the nervous system and minimize symptoms of anxiety. For example, The 4-7-8 breathing technique entails inhaling for the first four seconds, holding your breath for seven seconds, and exhaling for the next eight seconds. This exercise helps minimize stress and promote relaxation.

Progressive Muscle Relaxation

Progressive Muscle Relaxation (PMR) is a technique that is about tensing and then gradually relaxing different muscle groups throughout your body. This helps release physical tension and encourages relaxation. By focusing on the contrast between relaxation and tension, you can become more aware of bodily sensations and control overall stress levels.

1. Begin by tensing the muscles in your feet.

2. Hold the tension for a few seconds.

3. Now, slowly release the tension.

4. Gradually work your way up through your body, including the legs, abdomen, arms, and neck.

Time Management and Organization

Setting priorities: Effective time management can help lessen feelings of being overwhelmed. Prioritizing tasks, breaking them into small and manageable steps, and setting realistic goals can enhance productivity and reduce stress levels.

Organizing activities: Creating a to-do list or schedule can help manage responsibilities and make sure that enough time is allocated for both self-care and relaxation. Organization can also contribute to an enhanced sense of control and lower stress.

Creative Outlets

Engaging in hobbies: Pursuing hobbies as well as creative activities, such as writing, painting, or gardening, can offer a productive outlet to manage your stress and foster relaxation. Engaging in enjoyable activities also gives a sense of accomplishment as well as well-being.

Mindful activities: Activities that demand concentration and focus, such as crafts or puzzles, can offer a mental break from stress and help encourage relaxation.

Support Groups and Therapy

Support groups and therapy play an important role in managing the psychological and emotional challenges linked with perimenopause. They offer a platform for receiving guidance, sharing experiences, and finding solace in a supportive and friendly environment.

Benefits of Support Groups

- **Shared experiences:** Support groups provide a space where people experiencing perimenopause can share their stories, needs, experiences, and challenges. This mutual experience fosters an enhanced sense of understanding and minimizes feelings of isolation.

- **Emotional support:** Being part of a support group also offers emotional encouragement as well as reassurance. Members can give empathy and validation, helping others feel less alone in their struggles and challenges.

- **Information and resources:** Support groups often offer access to valuable information about perimenopause, including treatment options, lifestyle tips, and symptom management strategies. Members can also exchange practical advice and learn from each other's experiences.

- **Building connections:** Developing the bonds of friendships with others going through the same experiences can result in a supportive network. This connection can be a prime source of motivation and comfort throughout the perimenopausal transition.

- **Reduced stigma:** Engaging in support groups can help navigate and reduce the stigma during perimenopause. By frankly discussing experiences and symptoms, women can normalize their experiences and create a more positive outlook.

- **Online and in-person options:** Support groups can be in the form of both online and in-person meetings. Online forums as well as social media groups give you accessibility and flexibility, while in-person meetings offer face-to-face interaction and an enhanced sense of community.

- **Validation and empathy:** Engaging with peers and fellows who understand the physical and emotional impact of perimenopause can validate your feelings and cultivate a sense of empathy. This can be extremely important for managing feelings of frustration and isolation.

Types of Therapy

Individual therapy: These are one-on-one sessions with a therapist and allow for more personalized attention, guidance, and support. This approach is very useful for addressing specific emotional dilemmas and forming individualized coping strategies.

Group therapy: Group therapy sessions consist of multiple participants and emphasize mutual experiences and group dynamics. It offers a sense of community and unity along with gaining collective support. Moreover, there is always an added advantage of professional facilitation.

Couples therapy: Perimenopause can influence relationships negatively, and couples therapy can help partners deal with these changes together. It gives a safe space to communicate honestly and openly, address relationship issues, and strengthen the bond of partnership.

Psychiatric support: There are some cases when psychiatric support becomes a necessity to address a wide range of mental health concerns. Psychiatrists can prescribe medication and incorporate medical and therapeutic approaches for care and a comprehensive treatment plan.

Cognitive Behavioral Therapy (CBT): CBT is a commonly used approach that mainly focuses on recognizing and changing negative behaviors and thought patterns. It can be useful in managing symptoms of worry, depression, and anxiety during perimenopause by helping you cultivate and maintain coping skills and embrace positive thinking patterns.

Finding a therapist: When you are seeking therapy, it is crucial to explore different options so that you may find an experienced and qualified mental health professional who specializes in challenges and issues associated with perimenopause, mood swings, or women's health. Credentials, experience, certificates, and a therapeutic approach are the main factors to consider when you are selecting a therapist.

In a nutshell, support groups and therapy can offer you valuable resources for managing the psychological and emotional aspects of perimenopause. Moreover, regular sessions with your therapists and a balance between diet and exercise can help you mitigate the symptoms successfully.

Conclusion

The journey to getting to know the transitional yet totally natural phase of perimenopause has come to an end, and therefore, it is important that we review some of the most important points.

Perimenopause is a phase marked by uncertainty and significant change. It occurs in a woman's life anywhere between the mid-30s to early 40s and a woman experiences an irregular menstrual cycle. Its symptoms and intensity vary from individual to individual; however, common symptoms include constant fatigue, sleep issues, hot flashes, night sweats, and anxiety. The varying hormones can cause mood irritability and physical appearance also starts to change.

Although this phase is filled with emotional, physical, and mental challenges, you can navigate this transitional period with confidence and control by adopting the right set of strategies. The first step is to educate yourself about this phase and then understand your symptoms. This awareness and understanding allows you to understand that you can manage your symptoms and still enjoy your life. You realize that these transformations and shifts are a natural part of life and do not symbolize a loss of control or end of happiness.

Obviously, there are many factors that shape your perspective regarding this phase. For example, the cultural and social context in which perimenopause takes place greatly shapes a woman's experience. Societal attitudes, family dynamics, media portrayals, workplace settings, and social support systems all shape how women perceive and deal with this transitional phase. Identifying and addressing these effects can help you create a more supportive and nurturing environment for women, allowing them to manage perimenopause with enhanced resilience and a sense of empowerment.

It is by adopting healthy lifestyle habits, seeking social and professional support, choosing the right set of treatments, and managing your stress by employing various mindfulness techniques that you can mitigate the effects of hormonal fluctuations and sustain emotional well-being.

The significance of emotional support during perimenopause cannot be ignored. It plays an important role in strengthening relationships, fostering emotional stability, validating experiences, giving encouragement, and providing safe access to valuable resources. By having a strong support system, you can easily navigate the issues of perimenopause with grace.

Stress management techniques are vital for maintaining emotional well-being during perimenopause. Mindfulness, progressive muscle relaxation, regular physical activity, and deep breathing can help you reduce stress and improve your emotional health. Making healthy lifestyle choices persistently, building strong social bonds, and engaging in creative outlets further support stress reduction. By integrating these techniques into everyday life, you can better manage stress, anxiety, worry, and restlessness and improve your overall quality of life during this important and challenging phase of life.

Considering early retirement or a career change is a major decision impacted by the multifaceted challenges of perimenopause. The emotional, cognitive, and physical symptoms, merged into an unsupportive workplace and the need to re-assess your life priorities, drive a lot of women to seek new professional pathways or retire early. By comprehending these challenges, policymakers and employers can build a more supportive work environment to retain their valuable employees and assist women in navigating this phase with more ease.

Internalized ageism as well as shame also affect women experiencing perimenopause. These internalized beliefs, backed up by cultural norms and media, contribute to feelings of inadequacy, low self-esteem, and reduced self-worth. The result of these feelings can be seen in several aspects of life, from workplace dynamics to social interactions. Understanding and addressing this internalized ageism is of prime importance for supporting the mental well-being and physical health of perimenopausal women.

Raising awareness and promoting knowledge about perimenopause is also required to improve the well-being of women who are undergoing extreme symptoms. By bridging knowledge gaps, cultivating empathy, getting support for changing healthcare and workplace environments, addressing societal and cultural attitudes, and conducting research and policy development, we all can contribute to creating a more supportive, positive, and informed society. These efforts ensure that women experience perimenopause with the necessary support, dignity, and respect

With the passage of time, people, are becoming more aware of the challenges of this phase and the harmful effects of perimenopause. Media and people with influence are making a difference. The Hollywood actress Jennifer Aniston is among those celebrities who are talking about the issues and stigma regarding aging. In an interview, Jennifer Aniston discussed her own experiences with ageism and fitness in the context of not only her career but also public life. The actress, who is in her fifties, opened up about the societal expectations and pressures placed on women as they start to age. It has become a common practice that everyone thinks that women are supposed to look bad when they grow old. The actress has been told many times by people that she looks great when compared to her age giving the idea that "You should look like hell right now" (Denton, 2019).

Aniston reflected on how ageism appears in the media and the effect it has had on her, focusing on the challenge of maintaining a positive and healthy self-image amidst societal pressures and relentless scrutiny (Denton, 2019). She is not the only one affected by these stereotypes, thousands of women going through perimenopausal periods also feel the same.

Rather than letting society dictate or tell that you should hide or try to look more youthful, the actress suggests that no one should overlook the significance of self-care and wellness practices in their life (Denton, 2019). A lifelong commitment to well-being and fitness, which consists of a balanced diet, regular exercise, and a focus on mental health can help women navigate this phase with confidence rather than shame and embarrassment.

Moreover, know that health and wellness go beyond the world of physical appearance and involve nurturing your own mental and emotional health. You need to embrace aging with confidence and affection and that is how your efforts will contribute to changing the negative narratives prevailing in society toward aging and beauty.

Additionally, open communication with healthcare professionals can help you manage the complexities of perimenopause. It ensures accurate and on-time diagnosis, allows for customized treatment plans, addresses needs, preferences, and concerns, offers education, and fosters a nurturing relationship. By engaging in open and honest dialogue, women can navigate perimenopause with efficiency, receive appropriate care, and enjoy a better quality of life.

Last but not least, I am very thankful to each of you for staying with me until the end. Your commitment to reading this book is a testament to the reality that you want to enjoy a good life that results from maintaining good physical and mental health.

Our journey has come to an end and it is only a reminder that your own journey toward taking control over your health and life has just begun. Let the knowledge and strategies mentioned in *Navigating Perimenopause Challenges* guide you. At first, you may think *I cannot do it*, or *It is impossible to manage my symptoms*; know that if you have come so far, you can go ahead as well. Over time, you will see yourself dealing with this phase very comfortably. So, let patience and persistence be your friends.

If you have learned something new or if this book has helped you in any way, I request you to please leave a review, for your review can help others begin this journey with certainty and confidence.

May your journey be filled with ease and rewards!

Glossary

Ageism: Discrimination based on the age of a person.

Burnout: A state of physical, mental, and emotional exhaustion caused by prolonged and excessive stress.

Collagen: The main protein found in a human's body.

Empty Nest Syndrome: The feelings of emotional distress, grief, loneliness, or sadness that parents may experience when their children leave their homes.

Follicle-stimulating hormone (FSH): This hormone is involved in regulating ovarian function and the menstrual cycle.

Gender stereotypes: Preconceived ideas or notions about the behaviors and roles appropriate for men and women.

Hormonal volatility: Quick and unpredictable changes in hormone levels that can influence physical and emotional well-being.

Identity crisis: The period marked by confusion and uncertainty in which a person's sense of their own identity becomes doubtful and insecure, largely due to an important life change or stressor.

Luteinizing hormone (LH): This hormone works with FSH in the regulation of ovulation and the menstrual cycle.

Menorrhagia: Heavy menstrual bleeding.

Oligomenorrhea: Infrequent menstrual periods.

Oocyte: They are also known as egg cells. These cells are present in the ovaries and have the possibility to grow into a fertilized egg with sperm.

Ovarian follicles: The structures within the ovaries that keep and release eggs during ovulation.

Ovarian reserve: The total number of viable eggs remaining in the ovaries, which decreases with age and is a main factor in a woman's fertility.

Postpartum depression: A kind of depression that comes to the surface after childbirth. It owes some to hormonal changes and some to other factors. It causes severe anxiety, sadness, and worry for a long period after childbirth.

Sexism: Discrimination or prejudice based on a person's gender or sex.

Stigma: It can be defined as a mark of disgrace linked to a particular situation or circumstance, quality, or even a person.

References

Alblooshi, S., Taylor, M., & Gill, N. (2023, March). Does menopause elevate the risk for developing depression and anxiety? Results from a systematic review. *Australasian Psychiatry, 31*(2), 103985622311654. https://doi.org/10.1177/10398562231165439

Applewhite, A. (2014, November). *"Ageism is a cultural illness; it's not a personal illness." Frances McDormand.* This Chair Rocks. https://thischairrocks.com/2014/11/01/ageism-is-a-cultural-illness-its-not-a-personal-illness-frances-mcdormand/

The Blinkist Team. (2023, August 9). *15 Empathy quotes that will inspire kindness and understanding.* Blinkist Magazine. https://www.blinkist.com/magazine/posts/15-empathy-quotes-will-inspire-kindness-understanding

Bostani Khalesi, Z., Jafarzadeh-Kenarsari, F., Donyaei Mobarrez, Y., & Abedinzade, M. (2020). The impact of menopause on sexual function in women and their spouses. *African Health Sciences, 20*(4), 1979–1984. https://doi.org/10.4314/ahs.v20i4.56

Bougea, A., Despoti, A., & Vasilopoulos, E. (2020). Empty-nest-related psychosocial stress: Conceptual issues, future directions in economic crisis. *Psychiatriki, 30*(4), 329–338. https://doi.org/10.22365/jpsych.2019.304.329

Bromberger, J. T., & Kravitz, H. M. (2011). Mood and Menopause: Findings from the Study of Women's Health Across the Nation (SWAN) over ten years. *Obstetrics and Gynecology Clinics of North America, 38*(3), 609–625. https://doi.org/10.1016/j.ogc.2011.05.011

Canivenc-Lavier, M.-C., & Bennetau-Pelissero, C. (2023). Phytoestrogens and health effects. *Nutrients, 15*(2), 317. https://doi.org/10.3390/nu15020317

Cappelletti, M., & Wallen, K. (2016). Increasing women's sexual desire: The comparative effectiveness of estrogens and androgens. *Hormones and Behavior, 78,* 178–193. https://doi.org/10.1016/j.yhbeh.2015.11.003

Cherry, K. (2021, July 8). *What are neurotransmitters?* Verywell Mind. https://www.verywellmind.com/what-is-a-neurotransmitter-2795394

Chisholm, A. (2023, May 30). *Endometrial hyperplasia.* Verywell Health. https://www.verywellhealth.com/endometrial-hyperplasia-risk-factors-types-and-treatments-4067214

Cleveland Clinic. (2023). *SNRIs (Serotonin and Norepinephrine Reuptake Inhibitors).* Cleveland Clinic. https://my.clevelandclinic.org/health/treatments/2479 7-snri

Cowell, A. C., Gilmour, A., & Atkinson, D. (2024). Support mechanisms for women during menopause: Perspectives from social and professional structures. *Women, 4*(1), 53–72. https://doi.org/10.3390/women4010005

Denton, E. (2019, October 9). *Jennifer Aniston on the worst beauty decision she's ever made*. Allure. https://www.allure.com/story/jennifer-aniston-ageism-wellness-interview

Dhuli, K., Naureen, Z., Medori, M. C., Fioretti, F., Caruso, P., Perrone, M. A., Nodari, S., Manganotti, P., Xhufi, S., Bushati, M., Bozo, D., Connelly, S. T., Herbst, K. L., & Bertelli, M. (2022). Physical activity for health. *Journal of Preventive Medicine and Hygiene, 63*(2 Suppl 3), E150–E159. https://doi.org/10.15167/2421-4248/jpmh2022.63.2S3.2756

Erdélyi, A., Pálfi, E., Tűű, L., Nas, K., Szűcs, Z., Török, M., Jakab, A., & Várbíró, S. (2024). The importance of nutrition in menopause and perimenopause—A review. *Nutrients, 16*(1), 27. https://doi.org/10.3390/nu16010027

Exceed Hormone Specialists. (2015, May 4). *Top 7 quotes from women with hormone issues before menopause*. Exceed Hormone Specialists. https://exceedhs.com/blog/top-7-quotes-from-women-with-hormone-issues-before-menopause/

Galvan, J. (2020, June 17). *An Introduction*. Medium; Medium. https://medium.com/@jessgalvan8/an-introduction-c1bb2d5a1162

Grandey, A. A., Gabriel, A. S., & King, E. B. (2019). Tackling taboo topics: A review of the three Ms in Working women's lives. *Journal of Management, 46*(1), 7–35. https://doi.org/10.1177/0149206319857144

Greendale, G. A., Derby, C. A., & Maki, P. M. (2011). Perimenopause and cognition. *Obstetrics and Gynecology Clinics of North America, 38*(3), 519–535. https://doi.org/10.1016/j.ogc.2011.05.007

Harper-Harrison, G., & Shanahan, M. M. (2023, February 20). *Hormone replacement therapy.* National Library of Medicine; StatPearls Publishing. https://www.ncbi.nlm.nih.gov/books/NBK493191/

Harper, J. C., Phillips, S., Biswakarma, R., Yasmin, E., Saridogan, E., Radhakrishnan, S., C Davies, M., & Talaulikar, V. (2022). An online survey of perimenopausal women to determine their attitudes and knowledge of the menopause. *Women's Health, 18*(18), 174550572211068. https://doi.org/10.1177/17455057221106890

Harvey A. Friedman Center for Aging. (2023, March 28). *Internalized ageism – Discriminating against ourselves as we age.* Institute for Public Health. https://publichealth.wustl.edu/internalized-ageism-discriminating-against-ourselves-as-we-age/

Kong, J., Zhou, L., Li, X., & Ren, Q. (2023). Sleep disorders affect cognitive function in adults: an overview of systematic reviews and meta-analyses. *Sleep and Biological Rhythms.* https://doi.org/10.1007/s41105-022-00439-9

Lee, J., Han, Y., Cho, H. H., & Kim, M.-R. (2019). Sleep disorders and menopause. *Journal of Menopausal Medicine, 25*(2), 83–87. https://doi.org/10.6118/jmm.19192

Lee, Y.-J., Yi, S.-W., Ju, D.-H., Lee, S.-S., Sohn, W.-S., & Kim, I.-J. (2015). Correlation between postpartum depression and premenstrual dysphoric disorder: Single center study. *Obstetrics & Gynecology Science*, *58*(5), 353. https://doi.org/10.5468/ogs.2015.58.5.353

Marlin, D. (2017, April 21). *27 Quotes to change how you think about problems*. Entrepreneur. https://www.entrepreneur.com/leadership/27-quotes-to-change-how-you-think-about-problems/288957

Marques, P., Skorupskaite, K., George, J. T., & Anderson, R. A. (2018, June 19). *Physiology of GNRH and Gonadotropin Secretion*. Nih.gov; MDText.com, Inc. https://www.ncbi.nlm.nih.gov/books/NBK279070/

O'Neill, M., V. Faye Jones, & Reid, A. (2023). Impact of menopausal symptoms on work and careers: a cross-sectional study. *Occupational Medicine*, *73*(6), 332–338. https://doi.org/10.1093/occmed/kqad078

Qian, J., Sun, S., Wang, M., Sun, Y., Sun, X., Jevitt, C., & Yu, X. (2023). The effect of exercise intervention on improving sleep in menopausal women: a systematic review and meta-analysis. *Frontiers in Medicine*, *10*. https://doi.org/10.3389/fmed.2023.1092294

Schoenwald, C. (2024, January 25). *What I finally did after years of internal ageism*. The Ethel. https://www.aarpethel.com/fulfillment/what-i-finally-did-after-years-of-internal-ageism

Schulman, J. S. (2023). *Hypothalamus overview*. Healthline. https://www.healthline.com/human-body-maps/hypothalamus

Secomandi, L., Borghesan, M., Velarde, M., & Demaria, M. (2021). The role of cellular senescence in female reproductive aging and the potential for senotherapeutic interventions. *Human Reproduction Update*. https://doi.org/10.1093/humupd/dmab038

Sexton, C. (2022, March 28). *Menopause and anger toward husbands: The rage is real*. Mindset Health. https://www.mindsethealth.com/matter/menopause-and-anger-toward-husbands

Shiramizu, R. (2024, March 13). *How does menopause affect the body? Common symptoms & ways to help*. Life Flo; Life Flo. https://life-flo.com/blogs/news/how-does-menopause-affect-the-body-common-symptoms-ways-to-help

Thornton, M. J. (2013). Estrogens and aging skin. *Dermato-Endocrinology*, *5*(2), 264–270. https://doi.org/10.4161/derm.23872

Tredgold, G. (2016, August 4). *55 Inspiring quotes that show the power of emotional intelligence*. Inc; Inc. https://www.inc.com/gordon-tredgold/55-inspiring-quotes-that-show-the-importance-of-emotional-intelligence.html

WebMD Editorial Contributors. (2023, October 2). *What is perimenopause?* WebMD. https://www.webmd.com/menopause/guide-perimenopause

Wiginton, K. (2024, March 9). *Painful sex during menopause: What to know*. WebMD.

https://www.webmd.com/menopause/painful-sex-menopause

Women are 40% more likely to experience depression during the perimenopause. (2024). ScienceDaily. https://www.sciencedaily.com/releases/2024/05/2405 01091701.htm#:~:text=The%20researchers%20found% 20that%20perimenopausal

Worth, T. (2016, December 30). *SSRIs: Everything you need to know.* WebMD; WebMD. https://www.webmd.com/depression/ssris-myths-and-facts-about-antidepressants

Yeager, S. (2023, October 30). *What's the deal with shame and stigma about menopause?* Feisty Menopause. https://www.feistymenopause.com/blog/what-s-the-deal-with-shame-and-stigma-about-menopause